I0417472

YOUR CANCER NAVIGATOR

A Practical Guide for Your Cancer Journey

Betsy Murphy, RN

The information provided is not intended to be a substitute for the personalized professional advice given to you by a physician

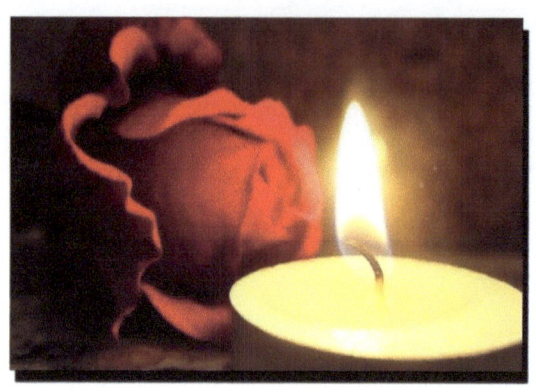

*Dedicated to all those that
lost the fight, and to those
who won't give up the fight.*

Table of Contents

Life was good. I know from experience that life can change in a heartbeat. One day I was fine, the next day I wasn't. I had found a lump.

Who do you tell? What do you say? Fear starts creeping in as I remember my Aunt Lovey and all the things she went through when she had breast cancer. Then there was a woman at church that's my age…she died from breast cancer. I was just thirty-four.

We all know someone who has, or had, cancer. Some are survivors, while others have suffered and that has helped build your perception of what cancer is.

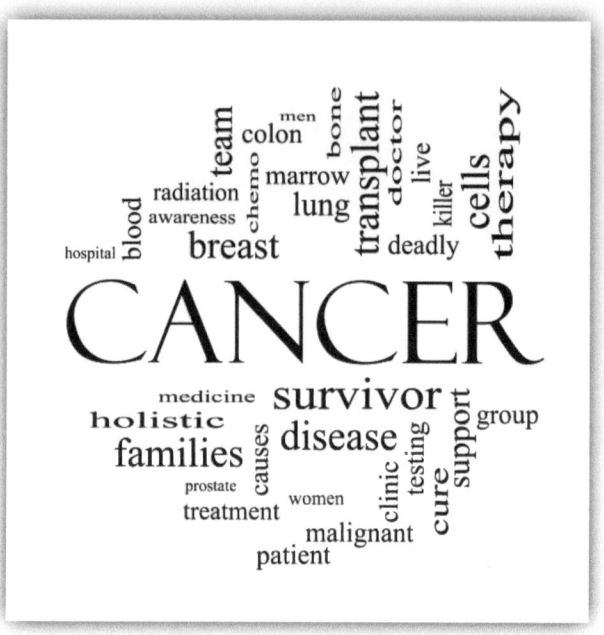

One thing is certain...even the thought of possibly having cancer is terrifying. Do not let your fear keep you from going to your doctor to be checked out. I know several people that have resisted going to see their doctor, because if they didn't know, then they didn't have to worry about it. That will not protect you. Early detection and treatment saves lives. Please don't hesitate and schedule an appointment. Your doctor would much rather see you and have your concerns addressed and cancer ruled out. If the doctor feels that there is a reason for concern, you found it early and your chance of survival is great. The last thing they want to tell you is "I'm sorry, but you have cancer, and wish you had come to see me sooner."

Cancer does not stop growing on it's own. It will continue to spread to various other parts of your body...the brain, lungs, colon, liver, etc. That is how cancer takes over and you lose the battle.

Be strong...be a fighter!

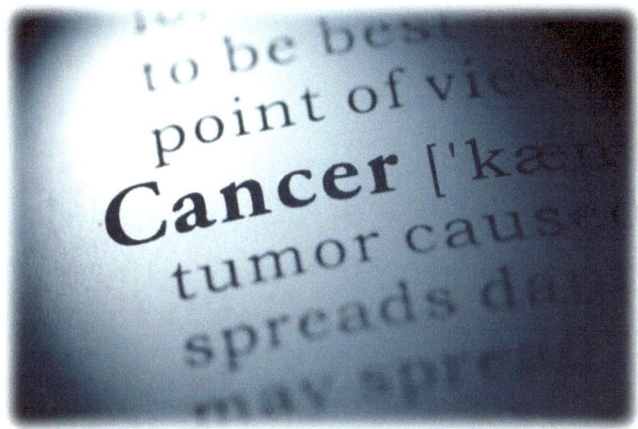

Diagnosis

You have had something show up on a scan...you most likely have had a biopsy. Your worst fear has come true...you have cancer. Take a deep breath. Your previous experience, if you have known someone and what they had to go through, will influence your perception as to what will happen with you. Clear your mind of preconceived notions because although there are similarities, we are all different. Your current state of health, pre-existing conditions, etc will determine your cancer treatment and how you will respond to that treatment.

Now you have the diagnosis, what happens now? All tumors are thoroughly examined by pathologist and a detailed report as to the type of cell, is it aggressive, etc. will be sent to your doctor. Your lymph nodes are biopsied as well. It is important to know if the cancer has spread beyond its original site. You will have further studies, CT scans of your chest, abdomen and pelvis.

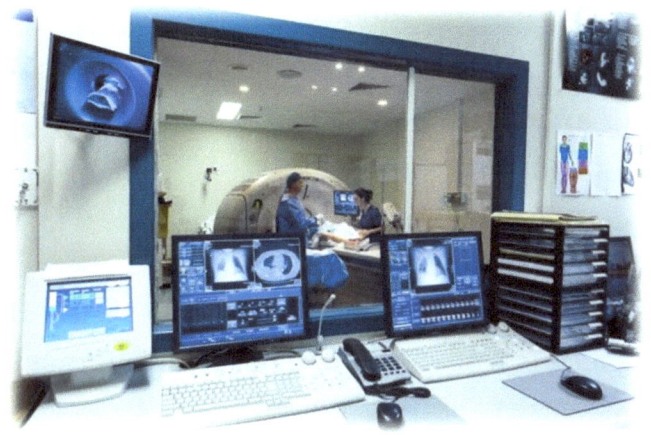

Also an MRI of the brain and possibly a bone scan will be scheduled for you. The ultimate test to determine a malignant tumor is a PET scan which is used when the other scans are not definitive. This will most likely be a very frustrating and stressful time for you. You get one test and have to wait on the results...then another test and wait on the results...it's maddening! When I had cancer the first time in 1992, it was so much easier. All the test have been completed as the doctor ordered them.

However, today the insurance companies dictate when the test can be done. Many times the doctors have to write the insurance companies if needed tests are denied. The insurance companies seem oblivious to the amount of stress we are experiencing and how they are making it much worse. So, just understand that this is a possibility.

Understand too that the time it takes to get your diagnosis will not be harmful to you. Your first thought will be "get it out!".   However, as I was always reminded, the tumor has been there for a while. The brief time needed to get your complete diagnosis is absolutely necessary.

Some of you will have feeling of grief from the loss of your appearance, loss of a breast, loss of the ability to maintain your active lifestyle, loss of a job and so forth. That's pretty common actually and many seek out counseling during this time. I went through counseling during my second cancer experience. I found it to be very helpful. Your cancer center may have someone available to you, or ask your doctor.

It's going to be important for you to learn some of the new terms. You may hear these at your initial appointment with your Oncologist, and throughout your treatment.

- **_Oncologist_**_:_ An Oncologist is a doctor that specializes in cancer care.
- **_Radiation Oncologist_**: Radiation Oncologists plan and prescribe the radiation treatments.
- **_Chemotherapy_**: A drug therapy that your Oncologist prescribes that uses powerful chemicals to kill cancer cells.
- **_Radiation_**: Radiation therapy treats cancer by using high energy waves to kill cancer cells.
- **_ADA_**: American with Disabilities Act: prohibits discrimination against people with disabilities in employment, transportation, public accommodation, communications, and governmental activities.
- **_Anxiety_**: A state of uneasiness and apprehension, as about future uncertainties. A cause of _anxiety_. A state of intense apprehension, uncertainty, and fear resulting

from the anticipation of a threatening event or situation, often to a degree that normal physical and psychological functioning is disrupted.

- **Cure**: Restoration of health; recovery from disease. A method or course of treatment used to restore health. An agent that restores health; a remedy.

- **Depression**: An illness that involves the body, mood, and thoughts and that affects the way a person eats, sleeps, feels about himself or herself, and thinks about things. *Depression* is not the same as a passing blue mood.

- **Chemo Brain**: a common term used by cancer survivors to describe thinking and memory problems that can occur after cancer treatment. *Chemo brain* can also be called *chemo* fog, *chemotherapy*-related cognitive impairment or cognitive dysfunction.

- **Late effects**: A health problem that occurs months or years after a disease is diagnosed or after treatment has ended. *Late* *effects* may be caused by cancer or cancer treatment.

- **Patient Navigator**: people who take individual *patients* through the continuum of healthcare as it pertains to their specific disease, ensuring that any and all barriers to that care are resolved and that each stage of care is as quick and seamless as possible

- **Rehabilitation**: a treatment or treatments designed to facilitate the process of recovery from injury, illness, or disease to as normal a condition as possible through therapy and education

- **Pre-existing**: any *condition* for which the patient has already received medical advice or treatment prior to enrollment in a new medical insurance plan, or medical treatment plan.

- **Primary cancer**: *defined* as the original site (organ or tissue) where a *cancer* began. For example, a *cancer* starting in the lungs is called *primary* lung *cancer*. If lung *cancer* spreads to the brain, it would be called *primary* lung *cancer* metastatic to the brain.

- **Metastatic cancer**: is cancer that has spread from the place where it first started to another place in the body.

- **Quality of Life**: that there is still purpose, enjoyment in life regardless of conditions, varies from person to person.

- **Recurrence**: Same type of cancer returns.

- **Remission**: A decrease in or disappearance of signs and symptoms of *cancer*. In partial *remission*, some, but not all, signs and symptoms of *cancer* have disappeared. In complete *remission*, all signs and symptoms of *cancer* have disappeared, although *cancer* still may be in the body.

- **Financial Counselor**: In the world of cancer care, financial counseling can benefit both providers and patients. Ideally, the process of financial counseling takes place with every patient, not only because it can help alleviate his or her concerns but because it can also help avoid unpaid bills. Honest, informative discussions about the financial aspects of their care empower patients by equipping them to take an active, informed role in their responsibility and overall treatment cost.

- ***Treatment team***: Everyone that is participating in your care. It includes physicians, nurses, radiology technicians, dietitians, psychologists, financial counselors...anyone else that assists in your care.

- ***Neutropenia***: the presence of abnormally few neutrophils in the blood, leading to increased susceptibility to infection. It is an undesirable side effect of some cancer treatments. It is a serious condition and may require hospitalization.

- ***Fatigue***: Extreme tiredness experienced during, and for perhaps a long time after, cancer treatments. Mostly caused from the effects the chemo has on the blood components. You may need blood transfusions if you have a low blood count, a main cause for fatigue.

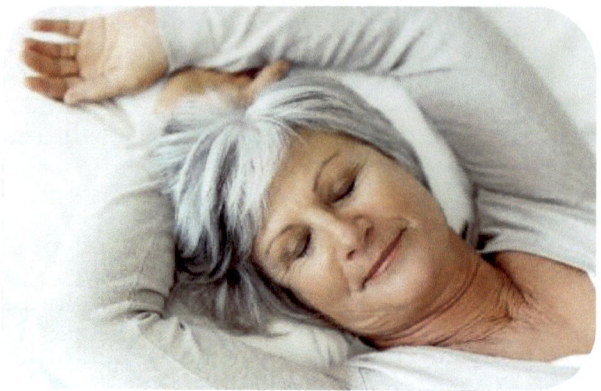

Choosing your doctor...

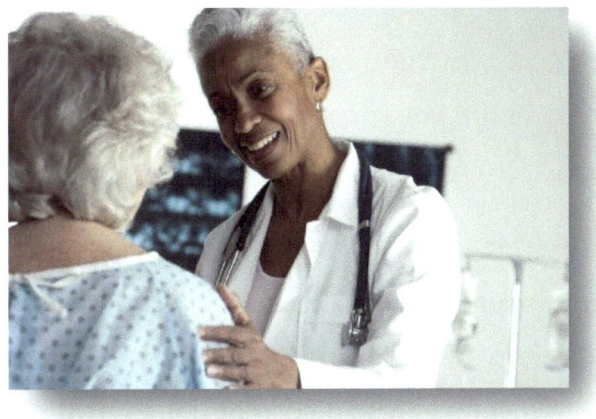

At this point you have determined something was wrong. You most likely saw your primary care physician for the complaint. The PCP then refers you to the surgeon, any surgery has been completed, and finally the referral to an Oncologist...your cancer doctor.

It is crucial that you trust your Oncologist, as well as the treatment he has planned for you. You need to feel confident that you received the best and the most appropriate treatment. Should you have a recurrence, or a new cancer crop up, you can feel that you did all that you could have done at the time.

Do you go with your local doctor, or go to a larger cancer center in another town? It is totally your choice. Again, you must have confidence in your cancer care.

However, there is something to consider. If you have a cancer that is better treated elsewhere, they would refer you to an Oncologist that specializes in that one certain cancer. The point is that all Oncologists are highly trained in their specialty. You might want to consider your hometown Doc for two reasons. Firstly, your support system is at home...you will need them. Secondly, the cost. Your cancer treatments are covered by your insurance regardless of facility. You will have multiple trips for treatments and doctor appointments. You may have to pay for motels and food. Cancer, is very expensive to treat and puts many into financial ruins.

I just wanted to make you aware as you are deciding on your treatment path. With all that being said, I can't stress enough that is it crucial that you are confident in your choices.

Once your friends and family find out about your diagnosis, they will want to rally around you and offer support. Don't be shy in accepting. You will find that others will want to do for you but not really know what to do.

Most will steer clear of talking to you about your diagnosis. They tell you, "oh, you're a fighter", or "you'll be fine", and so forth in attempts to make you feel better. Although they meant well, I felt they were blowing me off. I wanted to talk about my cancer and my treatment. I was scared...I wanted people to talk to me about fears, my not-so-good days, let me tell you about my treatments. I later realized that those that love you are scared too. Sometimes it was their fear that prevented the honest conversations that cancer patients long for. Tell those around you that it is ok to talk to you, in fact, you would appreciate it.

Perhaps you don't have family or friends nearby to offer you support. Your church family, local support groups, and co-workers. Don't be afraid to ask for help if you need it.

Treatment

Now that you've had your biopsy with the pathology report, any needed surgery and scans completed, it's time to see your Oncologist. You'll sign in and take a seat...you can't help but survey the others waiting for treatments or doctor appointments. You notice the wigs or scarves, a gentleman wears a surgical mask, a daughter helping her weakened mother into the waiting room. Nervousness increases as you wonder what will be your story, your journey.

Every appointment starts off with blood work. You'll be placed in the examining room. Your height/weight along with your vitals are charted, then you sit and wait on the doctor. It won't be unusual to just have a sick feeling being there, you want to be anywhere but here. For most, that feeling will never go away.

The moment has finally come that you meet your Oncologist. Your doctor will talk to you about the details of your pathology report. Treatment options will be discussed at this point. The choices are chemotherapy and/or radiation, hormone therapy, immunotherapy, or targeted therapy.

Surgery for some is all that is needed, and most likely has already been completed. Even if no treatment will be needed, anyone with a cancer diagnosis will still need to be seen and followed by an Oncologist.

You will have an exam by your physician. Oncologists are very thorough as they gather information about you, your current health. Pre-existing conditions will complete the assessment the doctor needs to plan your care.

For some it is difficult to decide to take the treatment while they feel fine. They feel that they should wait until they start having symptoms of the cancer...but then it is too late. It's important that it is your decision to take treatment or not.

What I tell folks, that want my opinion, that either way you are not going to feel well...either from the treatment or from the progression of the disease.

We already know the outcome of not taking treatment. If you are physically able to tolerate chemotherapy, I feel like you should try. If it turns out that you just can't do the treatment you can feel that you have done all that you can do.

Treatment is hard on you. When you are going through it, it seems it will never end...but it does.

Chemotherapy

Remember, chemo comes in different forms and selected based on your pathology report. Most of the time you will receive a combination of chemotherapy drugs...this is your *regiment.* It is referred to with a letter and is standardized so that any healthcare professional will know what the letters stand for.

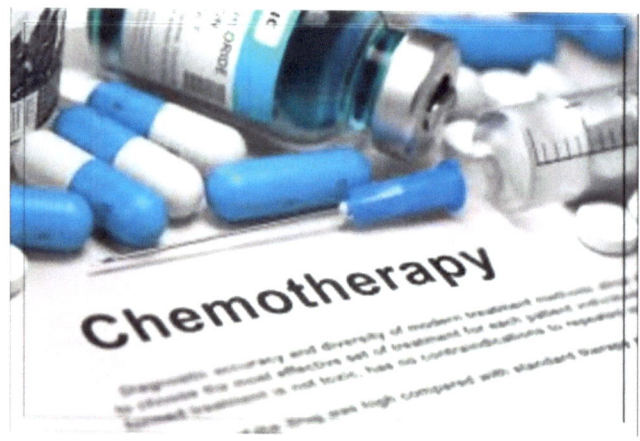

For example, one regiment I took was TCH.   That stands for the chemo drugs **T**axatere, **C**arboplatin, and **H**erceptin.

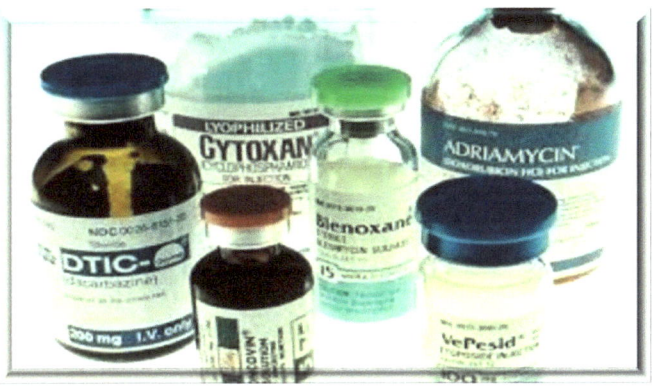

Some will choose homeopathic therapy. That is an alternative, natural approach to treatment. In my opinion, based on my professional experience, I do not feel that this is in your best interest. I have seen too many have tragic results with this course of treatment. In my opinion, it can help with your general well-being, but do not believe it can cure cancer.

I took care of a sixty-seven year old woman that had been diagnosed eight years prior with breast cancer. In getting her history, she told me that she had been adamant about not taking chemotherapy. She sought out various cancer doctors but they all recommended chemo for her and she'd move on to another doctor. She told me that she had done research and didn't find any evidence that chemo cured anyone. I thought I'd choke when she said that! She felt the chemo killed people. I told her my story...that I had breast cancer twice, had chemo, and had survived. I asked where she had gotten her information, but she wasn't able to tell me. She now was in excruciating pain as the cancer had spread to her spine, her lungs and liver. She is not going to survive.

The point to this story is that you need to make sure that the information you receive is accurate. Check you sources, talk with friends and if you choose to not take treatments, that is your choice.

As a nurse it was heartbreaking and frustrating to hear the woman's story knowing her decision was made on inaccurate information.

Treatment Begins

So now you're ready to begin treatment. I'm sure you have heard all the horror stories about the hair loss, the nausea and vomiting, etc. and are feeling pretty apprehensive right now. Well, some of that may be true. You most likely will experience the various side effects associated with the specific chemotherapy drugs you will be taking. Let me reassure you, **you can still have a life during your cancer treatment.**

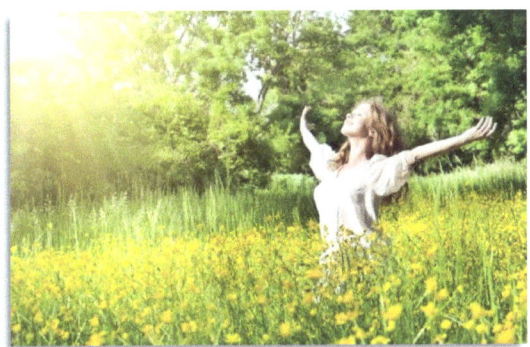

As you are going through your treatments, there are some things you need to know that perhaps you are not aware of. Let's start with the physical side of treatment since you are likely to have some knowledge of them. Talk to your Oncologist to understand what symptoms you might experience during your treatments. The way chemotherapy works is by attacking all cells which include the cancer cell. Unfortunately, it's the attacking of the normal cells that causes the side effects that you experience. If you are able research your cancer, your treatment regiment, etc to be as knowledgeable as you can. Always talk with your doctor and ask as many questions as you need.

It is important that you **do not** leave the doctor's office without understanding what you need to know. Everyone that works with cancer patients understands how stressed you are right now. It is ok to ask the same question multiple times if necessary. We know you are being bombarded with information and are feeling overwhelmed. Many feel that the doctor, or nurses, are too busy to be bothered with your question. That is not the case, we are never too busy for you.

Your treatments are done in cycles, meaning the time you receive your chemotherapy through to the next time you receive your treatment, is called a cycle. Cycles can vary, it's based on the drugs that are being used. Treatments are very structured in the way they are given. Perhaps you take treatments for two weeks and then off for two weeks, or your treatments are every three weeks. Just as predictable as the routine of the treatments, so will be the side effects that you will experience, and will be the same each subsequent cycle. You manage by treating the symptoms. Your oncologist will make sure you have what you need for nausea, pain, etc.

Each cycle consists of treatment time and recovery time. Just as regimented as the treatment, so are the side effects. If you start having nausea on day three following your treatment, you will have nausea begin on day three of the remaining treatments. You experience the same things, on the same days each cycle. Many worry about what's going to happen the next cycle, that it is totally unpredictable each cycle. I assure you that it is the same each time. It is because of that consistency of side effects that allows you to continue with your life as normal as possible.

Pay attention during your first cycle as to what side effects happen on what day, and how long they last. For instance, if you know that you start feeling queasy on day three, when you wake up on day three each cycle, you will start taking the Zofran the doctor has prescribed, just as prescribed, for the days you experience nausea. You will be able to keep ahead the game and keep the side effects to a minimum. Whatever the symptom, there is something that can help to keep you as comfortable as possible. Be sure to report all symptoms to your doctor so that they can help you manage those symptoms.

What is Your Treatment Like?

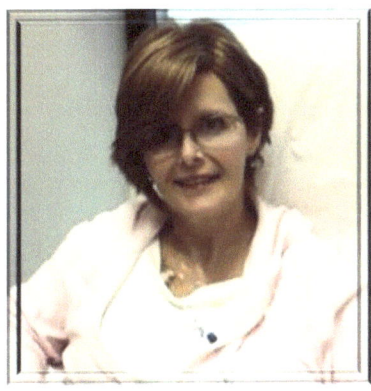

So, what will your chemotherapy day be like. Once you are called back to get your treatment, the nurse will access your Mediport or PICC line, or start an IV. They will draw some blood to make sure you are ok for your treatment. (If something is not right...your blood count is too low for instance; they will notify the doctor. They may have to correct the issue before starting your chemo.) Once everything is established that it's ok for your treatment to be given, your nurse will administer through your IV what is called your "pre-meds". Those are given before each treatment and most likely consist of the steroid to help lower your immune system, nausea medicine to help to keep the nausea at bay. There may be other meds given as prescribed by your physician. Once they are completed your chemotherapy will be delivered by the pharmacy. Your medication will be verified by two nurses as to the right person, the right medicine and the right doses before it is begun. Handling and administering chemotherapy is taken seriously and is very strict to maintain your safety, as well as the nurse. As you receive your chemo, it's just like a regular IV...you won't feel any difference.

Depending on your chemo regiment will determine how long your treatment will last. It might be an hour, or it could be five or more hours. Each treatment will be the same for each cycle. Dress warmly as it tends to be cool, and you may be feel a bit cold during treatment. You could bring a throw or the nurse can give you a blanket if you need it. You will be in a recliner and most facilities have individual TVs and magazines to help pass the time. You could bring some music to listen to and just relax. You may opt for just taking a nap. The staff will provide you will something to drink and snacks, so don't be shy about asking for something.

Side Effects...

You will receive information sheets on the drugs that you will be taking. Bear in mind that everything that could even remotely occur must be listed. Don't panic and think you will experience them all. *You won't!*

It can be overwhelming and frightening when you first look at the list of possible side effects. Let me tell you a little about them.

One side effect that not all will experience, but is one of the most frustrating, is *Chemo Brain*. That is the term for the mental fog that can impair your memory; your thinking. Take it from me, it can be maddening. You might experience things like:

- Forgetting things that they usually have no trouble recalling (memory lapses)
- Trouble concentrating (they can't focus on what they're doing, have a short attention span, may "space out")
- Trouble remembering details like names, dates, and sometimes larger events
- Trouble multi-tasking, like answering the phone while cooking, without losing track of

one task (they're less able to do more than one thing at a time)
- Taking longer to finish things (disorganized, slower thinking and processing)
- Trouble remembering common words (unable to find the right words to finish a sentence

Just be aware that this might happen, and may affect your ability to continue working or even various tasks in your everyday life.

I had to keep a little notepad with me... lists will be become your best friend. I got so I just laughed it off and didn't let it bother me.

From my experience, don't make any life changing decisions, your thinking and judgment may be impaired. I made some bad decisions before I realized it.

The main thing on most everyone's mind is hair loss. It will affect most people. Some may just have hair thinning and opt out of wearing a wig. The distress of hair loss is not just limited to us women; men also get upset about it. Emotions run from total acceptance and go bald, women with scarves, and men with hats. I have also seen the other extreme where the hair loss was more distressing than the treatment itself. You will need to prepare yourself for this. Even if your wig looks exactly like your hair, it won't look right to you. At first you will be self-conscience and think everyone is looking at you...they aren't. Your family and friends will see you bald and it will not bother them. They get used to your new look.

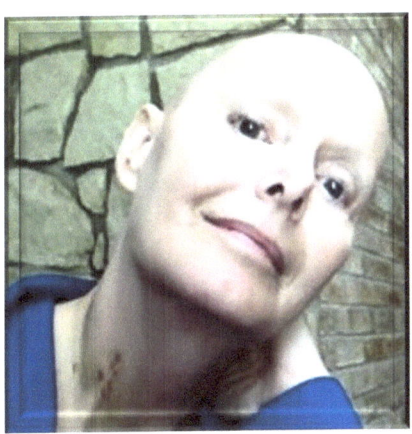

Here I am .. bald, no eye brows or eye lashes. My boyfriend still loved me and thought I was beautiful. His support helped give me peace of mind. I had experienced hair loss the first time, but not to this degree.

You need to get your wig as you are starting your treatment so you can get adjusted to your new look. You will be more comfortable wearing the wig out in public when it's necessary. How do you pick out a wig? First, check at your local American Cancer Society. They have new wigs that have been donated that you can get for free. If you choose to buy one, you should look for quality brands, such as Raquel Welch, Eva Gabor, etc. Many of those wigs are priced in the $120-$175 range. There are wigs that cost more but there are plenty of styles to fit your budget. The wigs will be synthetic, and I highly recommend that over human hair wigs.

I have not met anyone that has bought a human hair wig that has not regretted their decision. The synthetic wigs come pre-styled and are easy to care for. For them to look the most natural, choice a color that is frosted and don't comb them down flat. Style them by fluffing the wig. I have a video on my blog, www.yourcancernavigtor.com, to show you how to care for and style your wig, as well as the other tips I've mentioned here.

You wash them in a capful of Woolite and cool water. You don't need to buy special wig shampoo...save your money for something else. Once you have rinsed your wig in cool water, just take a towel and squeeze the water out. Shake it out and hang it upside down to dry.

It will look like a drowned rat, but don't worry, just shake it out and it's good as new. The style remains. Wash it every two to three weeks, more often if sweaty. Some wigs have special fibers that allows you to use a curling iron or flat iron on them to style as you wish. Make sure your wig is clearly marked as one that can withstand heat before applying any heat to it. Otherwise you will ruin your wig.

Another thing to consider is the cap construction of the wig. They are lightweight and vented to keep you cool. At the front hairline, you can get wigs with a soft felt fabric or with a lace front. The lace front allows you to wear your hair brushed back from your face without noticing it is a wig. It's a good idea if that's the way you normally wear your hair. However,

I have had both types of wigs and found the felt front wig lots more comfortable than the lace one. The term itself is misleading as it not really lace, it's more like a stiff piece of interfacing. It is very itchy, but decide for yourself.

You don't need to buy something special to put your wig on when you're not wearing it. Hang it from a door knob or bedpost, etc. allowing it to hang upside down like when you wash it. The crown is the first place they will break down. To keep in good shape don't just take it off and lay it down. The way it folds when you lay it down like that speeds up the breakdown of the crown.

You will feel self-conscientious. Trust me, with the wigs out today, no one, even someone standing behind you in the check-out line, will even notice.

Whatever you feel about it, it is ok. For those of you that will want to get a wig, let me give you some helpful tips. Your hair loss generally starts after the second cycle of your chemotherapy.

Chemotherapy affects your sense of taste, as well as the nausea. You may experience blisters in the mouth or esophagus, loss of saliva and so forth that will impact how well you can eat. There are a few things that can help do during this time.

Eat smaller, more frequent meals. That will be easier on your stomach. Limit the amount of what you drink at mealtime to allow the digestive juices do their thing. This will keep the indigestion, gas and diarrhea to a minimum. Drink plenty of fluids between meals. You may have to leave out the juices like orange, grapefruit and tomato to prevent heartburn or causing pain if you have blisters in your mouth.

Try not to lay down for a least an hour after you eat. If you must lie down, keep your upper body elevated on two to three pillows.

Your doctor may have you increase certain foods in your diet to help replace electrolytes and other nutrients that has been affected by your chemotherapy.

You will take over-the-counter medication to help with the diarrhea. You'll want to keep them handy and take with you when you go out.

For forty-eight hours after your chemo treatment, your urine is considered hazardous. Your chemo is filtered through your kidneys. If you are caring for someone that uses a bedside commode or bedpan, be sure to wear gloves when handling the urine. If you go to the bathroom in the toilet, you won't need to do anything special...just be sure to flush after each time you go.

Men and women will notice a change in their skin and make that an important thing to be aware of. Moisturize! Be sure to wear a high spf sunblock when out in the sun. Chemo will make you more sensitive and easy to burn. Take care of your hands and feet. With the dry skin, you skin can crack and become infected. The steroids you take as part of your treatment makes you more susceptible for infection. You may experience neuropathy (numbness and tingling sensation) in your fingers and feet. It can vary from being a nuisance to being very painful. There are medications to help relieve that kind of nerve pain, so talk with your oncologist.

Another symptom is fatigue. This is experienced by everyone at varying degrees. Know your limits, remember wherever you go, you have to get back. The first time I realized this I was at one end of the mall and my car was at the other! I thought I'd never make it back. This too can be managed by planning ahead for the tasks at hand. Learn to pace yourself and rest when necessary. One thing I found interesting is that with chemo you feel the overall fatigue, but if you take radiation treatment, they make you sleepy. You will have to take a nap every day after treatments. You may not be able to work while receiving radiation.

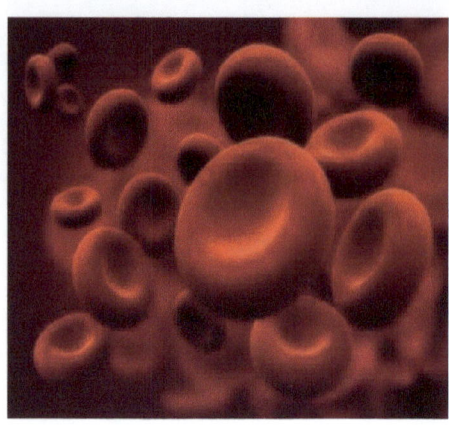

One side effect of chemotherapy that you may not notice, will be the effects on your blood cells. That means, it could be a lowering in the red blood cells that carry oxygen.

That will cause increased fatigue and heart palpitations and require you to receive a blood transfusion. Transfusions are done as an outpatient, like how you get your IV chemotherapy.

A couple complications you might encounter, low platelets and a decrease in neutrophils, that are serious enough that you most likely will be hospitalized until they are corrected. Platelets are a component of blood that helps blood to clot. There is a real risk of bleeding that could be life-threatening.

Low neutrophils will put you at risk for a life-threatening infection. These conditions are not taken lightly.

If you have low platelets you will not be able to shave…ladies that means your legs as well. You'll use a soft toothbrush so your gums won't bleed. You ladies in your child-bearing years could receive birth control pills to regulate your cycles so you don't experience a period during this time.

Neutropenia is a big deal. You will be taking a steroid during your treatments to lower your immunity so that the cancer cells are easier to kill. In addition, the chemotherapy lowers the neutrophils. If you should become neutropenic there will be precautions that need to be taken.

To give you an idea of how serious neutropenia is, I took care of a patient who was not able to leave the hospital to attend her husband's funeral.

You may encounter some challenges during and/or following treatment. Besides the physical side effects, you may experience depression or changes in your mood. That is normal and you will get back to feeling like yourself once it's over. The changes in the brain from the chemotherapy, the fatigue and illness can wear on you over time. It's easy to get discouraged...but DON'T!

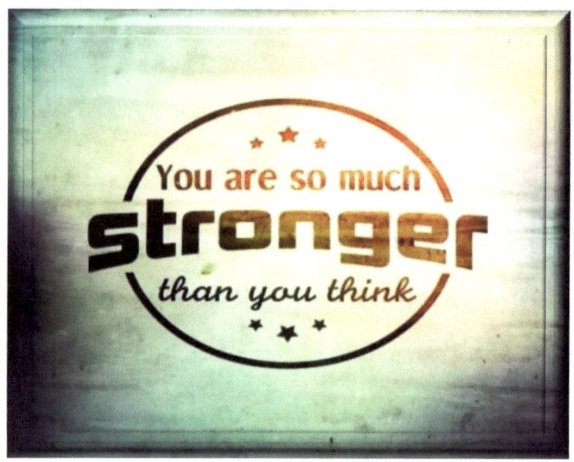

When you are going through all the unpleasantries it will feel like it will never end...but it does. Once you get through it all you will look in retrospect and realize it was just a short period of time. You have made it to the other side...

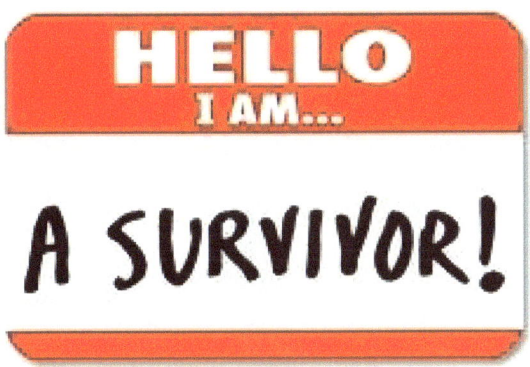

You will need to take extra care of your teeth. You may experience a dry mouth from your treatment and lends itself for extra bacteria to grow. You may not realize it until a year or so after the treatment's completion that you have cavities under the gum line. See your dentist and take preventative measures.

Relationships

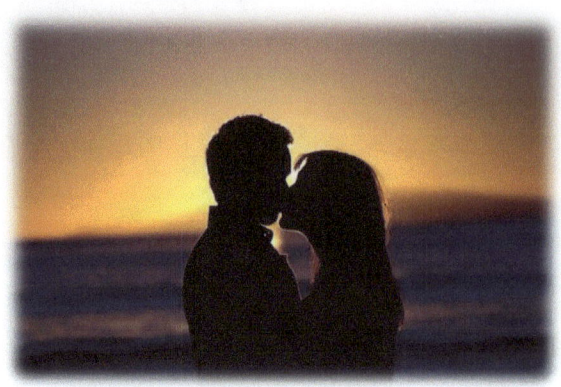

Cancer treatments and their side effects can affect relationships, intimacy and reproduction. Many couples turn together and their relationships become stronger. Many breast cancer patients feel disfigured and have expressed the lack of intimacy from their partner. Couple that with their own self-esteem issues and insecurities, that can wreak havoc in their relationships. On the other hand, many find their partners very accepting and supportive. Regardless of the type of cancer that you have, it is important to keep intimacy alive in your relationship. Yes, you are tired. Maybe you feel unattractive without your hair. The fact is that intimacy has a positive effect on your recovery. It has been proven that love, sex, cuddling and the like stimulates chemicals in our bodies to help us feel better. It is true that a hug can be good medicine.

If you young enough to still be planning your family, your cancer diagnosis doesn't necessarily mean you won't realize your dream of having children.

Talk with your physician. Some women will store their eggs until their chemo is over. That is done because chemo can cause infertility or damage the eggs and result in a very deformed baby.

Your Employer

You may or may not be able to work while you undergo your treatments. It will depend on the type of work you do, your health going into the treatments and the type of treatment you receive. The different chemotherapy drugs cause different side effects and their severity. I was able to work the full six months the first time I went through treatment, but couldn't the second time.

Hopefully you have an understanding and supportive boss should you need to take time off. However, some businesses may not be so helpful to accommodate you. The American with Disabilities Act protects you from employers and any actions taken against you for taking the needed time off for your treatment.

Furthermore, employers are required to accommodate you when you work, i.e.: longer breaks to rest, light duty, etc. You need to understand that should they terminate you, or make things hard for you because of your cancer treatments seek an attorney. Dismissing from your job is considered "wrongful termination" and you can sue them. I had this happen to me, and heard of others as well. Understand your rights that are protected by the ADA and stand up to your employer if necessary.

Cancer is expensive. You have the cost of treatment not covered by insurance, trips back and forth to doctor/treatment appointments, perhaps lost wages from missing work. The cost of it all sometimes can bring financial hardships. Where ever you receive your treatment, they will have a financial counselor there to help you. There are many sources of help available and you most likely know nothing of them.

When I was going the second breast cancer diagnosis, I was terminated by my employer. With that I lost my insurance. I was terrified! I thought I'd have to stop treatment until I was referred to the financial counselor.

She was able to enroll me into the West Virginia Breast & Cervical Cancer Program. It was a grant that provided me with a medical card that would cover all my cancer treatment needs. It was a lifesaver! If you have financial concerns during treatment, don't be too shy, or too proud, to ask for help.

Spiritual Well Being

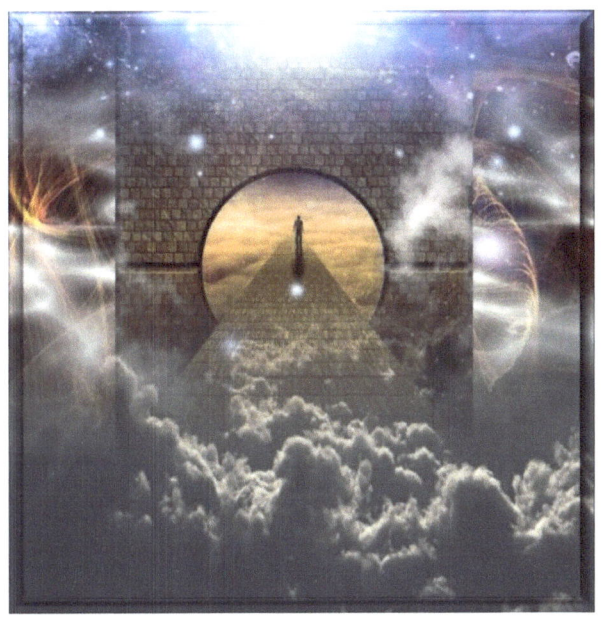

One source of comfort for many is prayer. Your spiritual life may be tested, (God why did you let this happen to me?) and it may be strengthened. Many turn to God during this time...have faith. God will be there for you. Even if you aren't a believer, there will be others praying for you. God hears those prayers as well.

After The Treatments Are Done

Ok, you have completed all your treatments...now what? You are eager to get back to normal. Well, it takes a bit of time to recover from all the effects of chemotherapy or radiation. Fatigue can last a year or two. If you experienced what is called "chemo brain" you may have some residual from that. I still have word-finding problems, I stumble over words at time, even processing thoughts. Don't be alarmed by side effects hanging around for a while. They diminish over time until you no longer experience them. Stay strong and don't get discouraged. You have fought a tough battle...give yourself time to heal.

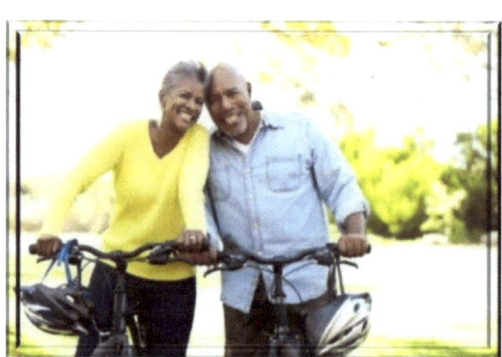

You may come out of this experience with a new focus on your health and the desire for a healthy lifestyle. Eating healthier, better food choices will help with you overall health. Dental health is very important. You may still have a dry mouth for a while after treatment starts, a breeding ground for bacteria causing cavities. Seek out things you enjoy doing and do them. Be with people that make you laugh. Mood boosters are always good, but especially now.

It is important for you to continue to follow up with your family doctor and your oncologist once your treatment is finished. You will continue to be followed by your oncologist, initially every three months for a year, then six months and then yearly. The oncologist will only monitor those things related to your cancer. You need to continue with you regular doctor for all your other care.

I can't stress enough that it is important for you to get in tune with your own body. Know what is normal for you and when something seems different don't hesitate to see your doctor. As you know, it is early detection that saves lives. Your doctor would rather you come in and have everything check out ok, than to have you wait and then your doctor has to give you bad news. No one knows your body like you. Once you have had cancer it is better to be cautious than sorry.

Even after treatment is completed and all is well, you will most likely keep cancer thoughts in the back of your mind. Twenty years had passed when I was diagnosed with breast cancer for the second time. I was a survivor for the second time.

You have to know your body, see your doctor when anything is out of the ordinary. It is just as important, if not more so, for early detection.

Cancer can take a toll on your body even if you tried to maintain strength and daily functions. You may need so help getting your strength back, full ranch of motion of an extremity after a mastectomy, and so forth. Your doctor may refer you to physical or occupational therapy. There is a lot you can do yourself like walking, exercising or even ballroom dancing. Find something you like to do that keeps you active. However, for some, just getting out of bed, bathing and dressing, normal daily activities may be difficult. Don't be hard on yourself, remember you may still feel fatigued for a year or two following your treatment. Give yourself time...you will get stronger, physically and mentally.

Questions you may have

Never hesitate to ask questions of your doctor and your chemotherapy nurses. Again, it is very important that you understand what they are telling you. Ask them to tell you again...as many times as necessary until you understand. We all understand that there is a lot to learn.

No one is too busy to spend time with you. Ask your questions.

- How did I get cancer?
- You say my cancer is in a stage? ... What does that mean?
- Should I get a second opinion before starting treatment?
- How do you know what treatment I'll have to have?
- What does chemo do to your body?
- What does radiation do to your body?
- Where do I go if I have questions?
- Will I still have symptoms after I finish treatments.

- Can I still have sex?
- What things should I avoid?

Resources

The American Cancer Society is an invaluable resource for about everything you'll need from being newly diagnosed, to recovery and beyond. They have educational information, to their various programs;

- Reach for Recovery

- Road for Recovery

- Look Good, Feel Better

- Relay for Life

- Hair loss & mastectomy products

There are many resources available and the American Cancer Society and/or the financial counselor at your cancer center to help get you started and help you make the connections you need.

You Did It!

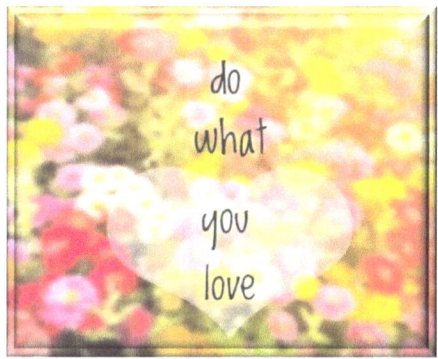

Undoubtedly you will be a different person once you finish your treatments. You will see life through different eyes. You will cherish even the smallest things, and every moment is not to be missed. Do things you've always wanted to do...take the trip, take the class, whatever it is...DO IT!

You will find that you run on a different clock than those who have not gone through what you have. You will realize you can't put things off, you will have a bucket list that you will compelled to fulfill.

Live your life to the fullest.

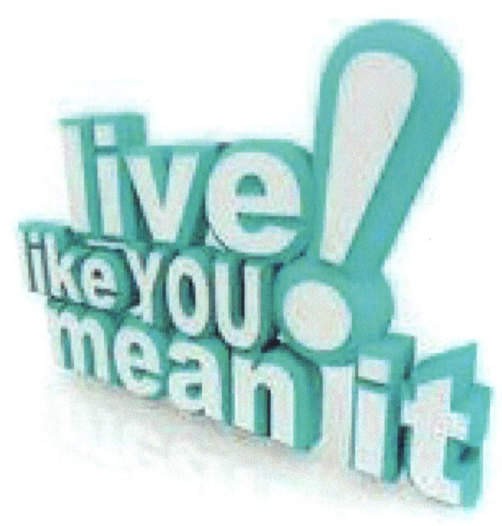

I hope you have found this helpful. I know that I was stressed and not knowing where to turn. Even though I was a nurse, I had never experienced anything like cancer. It is my hope that I can continue to help you by providing a blog where I post information that you will find helpful.

Everyone needs someone to turn to...I want to be that someone for you.

Visit my blog for ongoing education and tips to help you along your journey...

www.yourcancernavigator.com

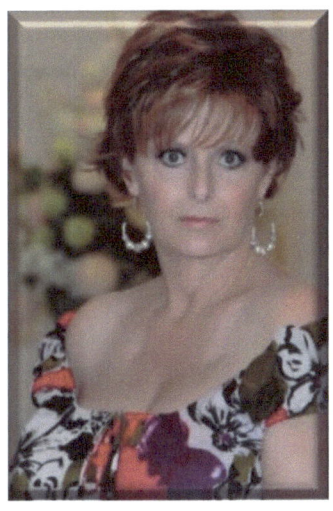

I wish you well. Be kind to yourself.

Betsy Murphy

www.ingramcontent.com/pod-product-compliance
Lightning Source LLC
Chambersburg PA
CBHW040325010626
45792CB00024B/2126